COLON HYDROTHERAPY

Alexis KOMENAN

COLON HYDROTHERAPY

ISBN 978-0-244-82972-8

Introduction

Colon hydrotherapy is a form of body hygiene and disease treatment that involves injecting water into the large intestine. Colonic hydrotherapy is one application of general hydrotherapy,[1] which includes oral water curing.[2] This therapeutic method, practiced since time immemorial, is undergoing a certain renewal, like natural medicine in general, especially among those who follow simple and natural health techniques.

However, colon hydrotherapy seems to be little known to the public and to classical medical science in particular. Some people disdain the method or even

---

[1] Hydrotherapy is the internal or external use of water, using various processes, for the relief and healing of ailments. The invigorating and healing properties of water have always been known to men, but hydrotherapy has been especially promoted by personalities such as Sebastian Kneipp, Vincenz Priessnitz, Simon Baruch, John Harvey Kellogg.

[2] The oral water cure aims to treat body aches and pains by cleaning the body and the large intestine in particular, using the large amount of water ingested. Although early morning water consumption upon awakening is a common practice in Asia, the scientific demonstration of the virtues of water cure has been established, according to a text reproduced by researcher Junji Takano, by a Japanese medical association (article available at the URL address: www.pyroenergen.com/articles/drinkwater.htm.)

reject it. Others find it virtuous and the followers of the cure say a lot of good things about it.

Therefore, we suggest that you go together to discover this method of health[3] that seems so worthy of interest.

---

[3] This small book is not a substitute for the health professional. It is recommended to also check with the competent medical authority.

I. What Is Colon Hydrotherapy?

The term "colon hydrotherapy" is made of two keywords: first the word "hydrotherapy," composed of two Greek terms, "hudôr" (water) and "therapeia" (care); then the word "colon," which refers to the large intestine.

Colon hydrotherapy is therefore the method of healing or restoring the shape of the large intestine by injecting water into it or, indirectly, by oral means. The technique is called "colon irrigation" in its long application and "enema" in its short application. In colonic hydrotherapy, water is used to stimulate, strip and disinfect the intestinal mucosa. But the beneficial action of the method goes beyond the single viscera treated to extend to the entire body, as we will see later on.

To fully understand colon hydrotherapy, it is first necessary to know, in a few words, the nature, the functioning of the large intestine and the properties of water, the ultimate healing agent of the method.

1. The Large Intestine

The large intestine is the last organ of the digestive system, after its companion the small intestine. It is divided into four segments: cecum, colon, rectum and anal canal. The colon is the most important segment of the large intestine since it makes up almost the entire size (1.50 to 1.80 m of ordinary measurement), so that the large intestine is often referred to, by extension, as the "colon." Its diameter varies from 3 to 8 cm depending on the parts, with a thick mucous membrane of 25 to 30 thousands of a millimeter.

The role of the large intestine is to receive the waste from digestion, store it and evacuate it through the rectal part (the anus), recover water and electrolytes, produce hormones,[4] ensure water balance[5] and absorb certain vitamins.[6] Some nutrients are ultimately absorbed at the organ level.[7] The muscular movements of the organ (peristalsis) control the whole process.

Performing such large functions requires state-of-the-art infrastructure and highly qualified personnel. To do

---

[4] The large intestine produces serotonin, or good mood hormone.

[5] It reabsorbs a significant quantity of water from the materials to be evacuated (about 86%) for the benefit of the body and regulates its quantity. Because of certain factors, excessive water reabsorption leads to constipation, insufficient reabsorption, diarrhea.

[6] This includes vitamin K2, produced by the bacterial activity of the colon.

[7] Jean Seignalet, *L'Alimentation ou la troisième médecine*, François-Xavier de Guibert, 5ᵉ édition refondue et augmentée, collection "Ecologie Humaine", 2004, p. 80.

this, the large intestine is populated by a multitude of "good germs" called the intestinal flora or the bacterial flora. This one is numerous and varied. These microbes are present in the mouth and are abundant in the intestines, especially in the colon. Surprisingly, the bacterial flora is more important in number than all the cells in the rest of the body.[8] It is responsible for all the functions assigned to the large intestine, this highly important central organ in the body.

The large intestine is mainly known for its role in the evacuation of waste products from digestion, also called feces or more commonly "stools." The specialists tell us that stool disposal is normally done one to three times a day. But, on the one hand, when several factors disrupt the proper functioning of the organ, such as an often inappropriate diet and lifestyle, the result is an accumulation of waste, fouling of the mucous membrane exceeding the "tolerable" threshold, resulting in pollution harmful to the intestinal flora and therefore to the entire body. This pollution is created by the poor disposal of waste, whose stubborn residues stick to the intestinal wall, ferment and release toxins into the bloodstream. On the other hand, the failure to occasionally maintain the organ, which would have made it possible to prevent and control the consequences of fouling, is a source of damage to the large intestine. All this makes up the favorable ground

---

[8] See for example O. Goulet, "La flore intestestinale: un monde vivant à préserver", *Journal de pédiatrie et de puériculture* (2009), 22: 102-106.

for multiplication and viral growth of microbes foreign to the normal intestinal flora. Specialists identify colon dysfunction, because of the volume of waste that is not drained and yet toxic to the body, as the source of many ailments and diseases of the body.

"The vital force will always seek to reject out of the blood as many toxins as possible. But what it cannot eliminate by the emunctories will be pushed back into the depths of the body. The toxins will thus penetrate to the inside of the cells. »[9]

Therefore, cleaning the excretory organ of waste par excellence by proper emptying is a guarantee of restoring its normal functioning. Such cleaning is an insurance policy against several conditions caused by the body's slow poisoning.

Water is therefore the right substance for this.

---

[9] Paul Carton, quoted by Dr. Jean Seignalet in *L'Alimentation ou la troisième médecine*, 2004, p. 339.

2. Water

Water, the "source of life," is a chemical compound found everywhere on Earth,[10] essential for all known living organisms. Water is the matrix of life, it is the living environment of most living beings.

Water exists in three forms: solid, liquid and gaseous. With the crude chemical formula H_2O,[11] water can dissolve over 80% of the known chemical elements.[12]

Biologically, plants are composed of 80% water and animals of an average of 65%.[13] The body of an adult human being is composed of 65% water on average, 75% in infants. The body's water is divided into intracellular water (about 60%) and extracellular water (about 40%).[14] Each of our cells contains 75 to 85% water.[15] The intracellular liquid itself is made of free water (95% of the total cellular water) and bound water (5% of the total cellular water).[16]

---

[10] The Earth is covered with 72% of its water, divided into surface water and groundwater.

[11] It was the French chemist Lavoisier who discovered the structure of water in 1785 and synthesized it from hydrogen and oxygen.

[12] See Jacques B. Boislève, *Structure et propriétés de l'eau*, 2010, available on the following website: www.sante-vivante.fr.

[13] See Daniel Robert, Brigitte Vian, *Eléments de biologie cellulaire*, Wolters Kluwer France, 2004, p. 20.

[14] See William McArdle, Frank I. Katch, Victor L. Katch, *Nutrition et performances sportives*, éditions De Boeck Supérieur, 2004, p. 78.

[15] See Eduardo D. P. de Robertis, E. M. F. de Robertis, *Biologie cellulaire et moléculaire*, Presses Université Laval, 1983, p. 82.

[16] Ibid.

Water occupies a unique place in the body. All functions are performed in the presence of water. The hydration of the body, so often neglected, is in fact essential.[17] Water provides nutrients, invigorates cells, filters, cleanses, purifies, detoxifies, regenerates, both in biology and in daily life, and in physiology, symbolism and spirituality. Water, the source and matrix of all organic life, is far from having revealed all its secrets to the scientific world.[18] It is one of the fundamental natural elements of old universal wisdom;[19] it provides the link, the communication, the synthesis between these elements.

Water "source of life," by its purifying nature, endowed with all its qualities, is therefore the ideal substance to restore life to the overworked or sick colon.

---

[17] See the work of Dr. Fereydoon Batmanghelidj and in particular his book *Your Body's Many Cries for Water*, published in 1992.

[18] Mohamed Larbi Bouguerra says: "In fact, liquid water is the most extraordinary substance we know. It is abnormal in all its physico-chemical properties. It is a unique product in its ability to exist, under normal conditions of temperature and pressure, in all three states of matter: gas, liquid and solid. This is the consequence of its particular chemical structure; moreover, it is not yet fully understood. " (in *Les batailles de l'eau*, p. 57)

[19] Ancient wisdom identifies the basic elements of the Universe: air, water, fire, earth. To which are added the wood and metal of the Chinese.

II. What Is the History of Colon Hydrotherapy?

Cleaning the intestines to maintain health is a hygienic and healing practice of a highly venerable antiquity.

Since the 16th century BC, indications relating to intestinal hygiene have been found in medical documents, the oldest currently preserved in the world: the Edwin Smith papyrus (1600 BC) and the Ebers papyrus (1550 BC). Many ancient peoples knew colonic cleaning,[20] reflecting an ancestral and universal medical wisdom from which all subsequent developments proceed. As proof, Indian Ayurveda, Chinese medicine and ancient Egyptian science include multiple indications for various conditions and methods of intestinal treatment.[21] In Greece, Hippocrates of Cos,

---

[20] See Charlotte Gerson, "A Short History of Enemas," *Gerson Health Newsletter*, Vol. 22, No. 2, March-April 2007, p. 1.

[21] See Chuan Zou et al., "Colon May Provide New Therapeutic Targets for Treatment of Chronic Kidney Disease with Chinese Medicine," *Chinese Journal of Integrative Medicine* 2013 Feb; (19) 2:86-91. We already have indications about enemas in ancient Egypt. In India, the method is called "basti" in Ayurvedic medicine. The American Indians have known about the cure since pre-Columbian times.

the doctor, describes intestinal cleansing and its benefits in the 5th century BC. Galen, in Rome, did the same in the 2nd century BC.

Then, intestinal hydrotherapy is commonly practiced in the small people and especially in the wealthy French classes of the Middle Ages, among other promoters are Ambroise Paré, the precursor of modern surgery (16th century)[22] and King Louis XIV (17th-18th centuries). But it was with the birth of the naturist and health reform movements of the 19th century and the early 20th century that the cure experienced a real revival of interest, in Europe with Sir Arbuthnot Lane and Professor Arnold Ehret among others, and especially in the United States with Drs John Tilden, Linda B. Hazzard, George W. Crile and John Harvey Kellogg among others. The great successes recorded by these practitioners, who studied the method scientifically, and its age, easily promoted its widespread use in the time's medicine. However, the second half of the 20th century marked the decline of intestinal hydrotherapy in hospitals, in favor of laxatives and surgery. But naturopathic medicine will mainly maintain this ancestral wisdom, with personalities such as Drs Bernard Jensen, Norman Walker, Victor Irons, Catherine Kousmine, Georges Monnier-Schraer, Christian Tal Schaller among others.

---

[22] See Christian Tal Schaller, *Hygiène intestinale: Retrouvez la santé avec un côlon dépollué*, éditions Lanore, 2006, p. 24.

Therapeutics is also experiencing a new, discreet youth in the West, particularly with the progression of so-called "soft" and "natural" medicine. Several scientific studies appear almost regularly on the subject.[23]

---

[23] See, for example, Douglas G. Richards et al., Colonic Irrigation: A Review of the Historical Controversy and the Potential for the Adverse Effects. *Journal of Alternative and Complementary Medicine* 2006, vol. 12, no. 4, p. 389-393; Yoko Uchiyama-Tanaka, The Influence of Colonic Irrigation on Human Intestinal Microbiota, *New Advances in the Basic and Clinical Gastroenterology*, Prof. Tomasz Brzozowski (Ed.), 2012.

III. What Are the Procedure and Mechanism for Colon Cleansing?

Whatever the method adopted, anal or oral, the common aim is to stimulate the large intestine to return to the normal physiological rhythm of waste disposal, beneficial to the whole body.

Anal colon hydrotherapy requires a minimum of water injection equipment in the large intestine. Different equipments were used for rectal hydrotherapy, but all have in common they are adapted to the physiology of the large intestine. Among the peoples of Antiquity - and even until now in some places - stems, vines and gourds were used by emptying their contents to serve as containers.[24] Animal horns were even used.[25] In the West, the era of the clyster syringe, popular in the Middle Ages,[26] was followed by the bulb syringe in the 19th century, to which were added bocks, pumps and

---

[24] The Enema - Heir to the Clyster, *S. A. Medical Journal*, 1947.
[25] See for example Katalin Cziranku, *Colon Hydrotherapy Is a [Scientificaly] Sound and [Medicaly] Valid Healing Modality*, PowerPoint presentation available at www.colon-therapy.org.
[26] See Christian Tal Schaller, op. cit.

dual-purpose cannulas. Elsewhere, traditional intestinal drainage procedures are maintained, but over time, they are often replaced by more "modern" equipment such as the bulb syringe or rubber enema pear, so familiar to mothers in sub-Saharan Africa.

As for the operating mode itself, it is generally conducted, with a few differences, as follows:

1. Taking an appropriate position (either in a curved or kneeling position, or lying on your right side according to some specialists).

2. The delicate introduction of the tip of the instillation material (pear, cannula, etc.) into the rectum (anus).

3. Irrigation of the colon with the introduced water, with delicate alternation of the irrigation flow, and accompanied if required by a small massage to stimulate peristaltic movements of the intestine and thus promote the complete evacuation of toxic residues.

4. The removal of waste so pursued, alternating with the instillation of water, by natural colon movement, or by stimulated movement (for example, sitting in the toilet and waiting).

It is also important to note that other adjuvant substances that are highly beneficial for the cure can be added to the colon draining water, which will be warm or cold[27] as needed: infusions and decoctions of

---

[27] Ibid.

indicated medicinal plants,[28] fine dietary clay powder in prescribed quantities,[29] good quality human urine,[30] sea salt,[31] natural ground coffee,[32] etc.

Before cleaning the large intestine, it is advisable to know its complete state of health to avoid contraindications (for example with advanced pregnancy or severe hemorrhoids) or adapt the treatment accordingly.

As measures to be taken to put all the chances on your side, it will be ensured that the room of the session (shower room, WC, hospital room) and the related equipment are healthy. We can never insist enough on the cleanliness of the premises and tools. The ideal time to cleanse your colon is when you are most free, such

---

[28] Dr. William Lieberman, an American specialist, saw warm water and salt as the best ingredients for an enema (in Enemas - Heirs to the Clysters, op. cit. p. 279). Dr. Paul Carton (in Edouard Bertholet, *Le retour à la santé et à la vie saine par le jeûne*) cites a book, *Les vertus médicinales de l'eau commune ou recueil des meilleures pièces qui ont été écrites sur cette matière* (Paris, 1730). It mentions ice-water enemas given to patients by Father Bernard of Malta in the early 18th century.

[29] See Christian Tal Schaller, *Hygiène intestinale : retrouver la santé avec un côlon dépollué*, éditions Lanore, 2006, p. 99 ; Roger Groos, Modern Naturopathic Colonic Hydrotherapy, *Complementary and Alternative Medicine magazine*, 2010 Aug: 12.

[30] See Dr. Soleil, *Amaroli, Source de Vie*, éditions Vivez Soleil, 1990, p. 18.

[31] See Jean Pliya, *Comment retrouver la forme*, éditions Les classiques africains, coll. "Les petits guides de la santé naturelle", 1996, p. 19.

[32] Dr. Max Gerson has used this adjuvant particularly in his naturist treatment of cancer through the intestinal tract. The liver is, according to its method, the main organ targeted by this treatment.

as on weekends or during school or professional vacations.

For the conduct of the cure itself, a certain experience of the practitioner in this matter, however simple the method, is essential, failing which it will be necessary to seek the help of a doctor specialized in the cure. This is particularly the case for the water-intensive irrigation technique. As for the enema, you can administer it yourself. Children of a certain age will of course be administered the enema by their mothers, as has always been the case.

A preparation of the digestive system the day before or a few days before is the ideal way to undergo it. This is done by a diet, at dinner the day before the session, not too copious, ideally made of fresh fruit and vegetables mostly, and preferably light. Hygieno-dietary improvement is important for the aftercare.

Submission to a fasting colonic irrigation session (abstention from food before the cure), without being necessary, is, according to the general opinion of specialists, recommended. Moreover, hydrotherapy is often associated with therapeutic fasting, with which it forms an explosive duo in naturist cures. The amount of water used per session varies according to people's appreciation and whether enema or flushing is performed. The same goes for the duration, which is essentially a function of each person's occupations and wishes. The same applies to the frequency, which we would like to be reasonable, and which depends on the biology of the organism, the needs, the appreciation of individuals and the doctor. It is always wise to take into account the opinion of the latter.

The water thus introduced into the intestinal tube will stimulate the wall of the large intestine, soften the waste (for the most persistent several sessions are necessary), thus preparing its evacuation. The practitioner's small muscular movements, even on the abdomen, and his expert and delicate massages also help the task. Colon cleansing also stimulates other emunctories and cleanses "all areas of weakness in the body."[33]

For oral hydrotherapy, it is a matter of drinking, according to the source, a quantity of water from 0.25 to 1 liter, depending on your age and weight, over a certain period,[34] from 3 to 90 days depending on your needs. The cure is used in the morning upon awakening, on an empty stomach, and can be adapted for beginners. This ensures a decongestion of the digestive organs, a good evacuation of waste because of the pressure of the volume of water in the colon as well as a more general cleaning via the body's emunctories.

---

[33] See Vincent Delaveyne, "L'hydrothérapie du colon", p. 3, available at the following URL address: www.iphosante.com/hdc.pdf.
[34] See Junji Takano's reference at www.pyroenergen.com/articles/drinkwater.htm and Dr. Batmanghelidj's work (website: www.watercure.com).

from ankylosing spondylitis[41] thanks to a naturist treatment including colon irrigation.[42]

Nevertheless, the method, especially in its long application, is still strongly welcomed with reservation, when it is not refuted, within the medical community itself.[43] W. Alvarez, at the beginning of the 20th century, then Dr. Edzard Ernst among others, put forward the scientific invalidity of the theory of self-intoxication, an essential postulate for the legitimacy of intestinal hydrotherapy.[44] Other studies focus on the possible disadvantages of the treatment, particularly on the integrity of the intestinal membrane and the risks of infection.[45] But all practitioners of the method,

---

[41] Ankylosing spondylitis, also known as Bekhterew-Marie-Strümpell disease, is a serious arthritic condition.

[42] See Dr. Irons' website: www.veirons.com.

[43] See Edzard Ernst, Colonic Irrigation and the Theory of Autointoxication: A Triumph of Ignorance over Science. *J. Clin. Gastroenterol.* 1997; 24:196-198; Ranit Mishori, Aye Otubu, Aminah Alleyne Jones, The Dangers of Colon Cleansing, *The Journal of Family Practice* 2011, vol.60, no. 8; Colon Therapy/Colonic Irrigation. Natural Standard Professional Monograph. 2011. Available at: http://naturalstandard.com/databases/hw/colon.asp.

[44] See W.C. Alvarez, Origin of the So-Called Autointoxication Symptoms, *Journal of American Medicine Association* 1919; 72: 8-13; Edzard Ernst, op. cit.

[45] See for example M. P. Tan, D. M. Cheong, Life-Threatening Perineal Gangrene from Rectal Perforation Following Colonic Hydrotherapy: A Case Report. *Annals of Academy of Medicine of Singapore* 1999; 28 (4): 583-5; D. V. Handley, N. A. Rieger, D. J. Rodda, Rectal Perforation from Colonic Irrigation Administrated by Alternative Practitioners. *Med. J. Aut.* 2004; 181 (10): 575-6; N. Ratnaraja, N. Raymond, Extensive Abscesses Following Colonic Hydrotherapy. *Lancet Infect. Dis.* 2005; 5 (8):527; G.R. Istre et al., An Outbreak of Amebiasis Spread by Colonic Irrigation at a Chiropractic Clinic.

scientists or ordinary people, agree to recognize the high tonic and healing virtues of colon hydrotherapy, provided that the treatment is carried out with tact and practiced with all the required rationality.

New England Journal of Medicine 1982; 307 (6): 339-42; F. Seow-Choen, The Physiology of Colonic Hydrotherapy. *Colorectal Diseases* 2009;11 (7):686-8.

Conclusion

Colon hydrotherapy was born largely out of the need to revitalize or cure the large intestine overloaded with toxic substances, because of an often denatured diet and a lack of maintenance of this highly strategic organ for health.

This exploration of the world of colon hydrotherapy has allowed us to appreciate the importance of this method of health for humanity.

We have found this practice since ancient times, from the immemorial peoples of history to the first great civilizations. Maintaining the large intestine has always been universally recognized throughout history as a key factor in health, physical and even mental well-being. In such a context, the invention and popularization of methods of short enemas or flushing of the large intestine have emerged as a social reality at one time or another in domestic life.

The effectiveness of colon hydrotherapy methods in preventing or treating many ailments, alone or in combination with other natural therapies, is further confirmed by several scientific studies. Examples abound in this work.

As with anybody care technique, essential knowledge and control combined with reasonable use of the method is necessary to achieve the greatest benefits from colon hydrotherapy. While intestinal cleansing is one of the most affordable methods of health, we should always take wise precautions to achieve the desired effect and avoid harmful errors at the same time.

While anal intestinal hydrotherapy was the main part of our discussion, we cannot conclude without reminding the reader of the importance of the other variant of colonic cleansing, oral hydrotherapy, commonly referred to as "water cure." Although indirect and therefore less instantaneous than the anal method, oral hydrotherapy remains undoubtedly one of the most effective, economical and easy-to-undertake health measures. This is for a few good sips of water taken successively over time - with no other equipment than a drinking vessel.

Finally, it is beneficial to keep in mind that colon hydrotherapy must be part of a more general desire to reform the individual's overall health habits. As far as possible, we will pay greater attention to physical nutrition, which should be healthier and more natural, and to psychological and spiritual nutrition.

We strongly encourage the public and health professionals in particular to take an interest in colon hydrotherapy, this thousand-year-old health method, so accessible and so capable of saving so many precious human lives, many of which are so often lost because of our ignorance.

Peace and Health to all!

Bibliography

CHURCH, J. M., Warm Water Irrigation for Dealing with Spasm during Colonoscopy: Simple, Inexpensive and Effective, *Gastrointest. Endosc.* 2002 Nov; 56 (5): 672-4.

ERNST, Edzard, Colonic Irrigation and the Theory of Autointoxication: A Triumph of Ignorance over Science, *Journal of Clinical Gastroenterology*, 1997 June; 24 (4): 196-8.

ERNST, Edzard, Colonic Irrigation: Therapeutic Claims by Professional Organisations, A Review, *Int. J. Clin. Pract.* March 2010, 64-4, 429-431.

GROOS, Roger, Modern Naturopathic Colonic Hydrotherapy, *Complementary and Alternative Medicine Magazine*, 2010 Aug: 12.

JENSEN, Bernard, *Tissue Cleansing Through Bowel Management*, BJ Enterprises, USA, 1981.

JENSEN, Bernard, *Dr. Jensen's Guide to Better Bowel Care*, Avery, USA, 1999.

KELLOGG, John H., *Rational Hydrotherapy*, 1903, reprinting Kiessinger Publishing, 2003.

KELLOGG, John H., *Autointoxication or Intestinal Toxemia*, Modern Medical Publishing Co, 1922.

KNOX, J. Glen, Enemas and Colonics, *Health Freedom News*, Jan 1990: 38-44.

LANE, William A., Some Remarks on Chronic Intestinal Stasis, *Lancet*, 1918, Sept 28, p.416-7.

MONNIER-SCHRAER, Georges, *La santé par l'hygiène intestinale*, éditions Jouvence, 2001.

RICHARDS, Douglas G., et al., Colonic Irrigation: A Review of the Historical Controversy and the Potential for Adverse Effects, *Journal of Alternative and Complementary Medicine* 2006 May; 12 (4) 389-93.

SCHALLER, Christian T., *Hygiène intestinale : retrouvez la santé avec un côlon dépollué*, éditions Lanore, 2006.

UCHIYAMA-TANAKA, Y., Colon Irrigation Causes Lymphocyte Movement from Gut-Associated Lymphatic Tissues to Peripheral Blood, *Biomedical Ress.* 2009 Oct; 30 (5) 311-4.

UCHIYAMA-TANAKA, Y., The Influence of Colonic Irrigation on Human Intestinal Microbiota, *New Advances in the Basic and Clinical Gastroenterology*, Prof. Tomasz Brzozowski (Ed.), 2012.

WALKER, Norman W., *Colon Health*, Norwalk Press, Arizona, 1979.

ZOU, Chuan, et al., Colon May Provide New Therapeutic Targets for Treatment of Chronic Kidney Disease with Chinese Medicine, *Chinese Journal of Integrative Medicine* 2013 Feb; (19) 2: 86-91.

Table of Contents